A DEMENTIA CAREGIVER'S GUIDE TO CARE
Frequently Asked Questions

Dr. Macie P. Smith
Licensed Gerontology Social Worker

©2019 Dr. Macie P. Smith Publishing
Columbia, SC

Copyright© 2019 by Dr. Macie P. Smith Columbia, SC 29201

All rights reserved. You may print, reproduce, retrieve, or use the information and images contained in this book for non-commercial, personal, or educational purposes only, provided that you (1) do not modify such information and (2) include both this notice and any copyright notice originally included with such information. If material is used for other purposes, you must obtain prior written permission from Dr. Macie P. Smith to use the copyrighted material prior to its use.

The opinions and views uniquely expressed in this book are that of Dr. Macie P. Smith based on her years of research and experience, both professionally and personally and should not be used in lieu of medical care or medical advice. The information in this book is not intended to be a substitute for professional medical advice, diagnosis, or treatment. Always seek the advice of your physician or other qualified health providers with any questions you may have regarding a medical condition. Never disregard professional medical advice or delay in seeking it because of something you have read in this book. If you think you may have a medical emergency, call your doctor or 911 immediately.

Dr. Macie P. Smith does not recommend or endorse any specific tests, physicians, products, procedures, opinions, or other information that may be mentioned in this book. Reliance on any information provided by Dr. Macie P. Smith, Dr. Smith's employees, others contributing to this book at the invitation of Dr. Smith, or other patrons of this book is solely at your own risk. In no event shall Dr. Macie P. Smith, her content providers, her suppliers, or any third parties mentioned in this book be liable for any claims or damages (including, without limitation, direct, incidental and consequential damages, personal injury/wrongful death, or lost profits) resulting from the use of or inability to use the information in this book, whether based on warranty, contract, tort, or any other legal theory, and whether or not Dr. Macie P. Smith is advised of the possibility of such damages.

Dedication

To my number one fan, my devoted husband, Marlon J. Smith. Thank you honey for always saying yes! I love you. To my nine-year old daughter, Mirah J. Smith, thank you, sweetie pie, for always encouraging my learning and my growth while working with the aging population. You always say to me "Mommy, you can stay with me and my husband. I'll take care of you." That is music to my ears. Thank you, baby!

To my A-team, my OnPoint Media team, thank you for your trust, support, and friendship over the years. I applaud you for stepping out on faith and seeing beyond what others see in order to change the face of aging and to offer a constant resource for seniors and their families . Thank you for your time, talent, and your innate ability to trust the process. This one's for you.

To my mom and dad, you always kept me grounded and humbled through my journey. Thank you for being my parents, not some of the time, but all of the time. The foundation you established for me is unwavering and for that, "thank you" will never be enough. It is because of both of you that I stand here today. I love you!

In loving memory of my sweet, sweet grandma, Mildred Perry. She fought a masterful fight and taught me a lot along the way about how to care for the soul of a person living with Alzheimer's. And now I get to share with the world. Sleep in peace my precious gem.

"Dear friend, I pray that you may enjoy good health and that all may go well with you, even as your soul is getting along well."

3 John 1:2

foreword

by

James T. McLawhorn Jr.

As the President & CEO of the Columbia Urban League, I am honored to write this foreword for Dr. Macie Smith's guidebook on dementia. Several years ago, Dr. Smith joined the Columbia Urban League as a consultant to empower African American and other underserved communities that were adversely affected by Alzheimer's disease and dementia. Since its inception in 1967, the Columbia Urban League has been at the forefront of empowering communities and changing lives through service delivery, advocacy and bridge building. The Columbia Urban League has over 50 years of empowering African American and other underserved communities to secure self-reliance in education, employment, and economic development and promoting healthy and safe communities to eliminate health disparities. I was pleased to support Dr. Smith's efforts in addressing the growing needs of family caregivers who care for those living with dementia. She has educated and trained hundreds of dementia caregivers in South Carolina as well as across the country.

I have seen the impact Dr. Smith's dementia education has had on families. Because of her innate ability and passion to present complex ideas in a dementia-friendly capacity, family caregivers have reported that their stress levels have decreased tremendously after learning practical ways to manage the care of their loved ones. After reading this guidebook, I am certain you will find comfort, support, and a new outlook on dementia- capable practices.

foreword

by

Cynthia Pryor Hardy

According to the AARP, 10,000 baby boomers are turning 65 every single day, and this is expected to continue into the 2030s. This means that nearly seven baby boomers are turning 65 every minute.

The aging of the baby boom generation could fuel a 75 percent increase in the number of Americans needing caregivers or requiring nursing home care, to about 2.3 million in 2030 from 1.3 million in 2010. The demand for elder care will also be fueled by a steep rise in the number of Americans living with Alzheimer's disease, which by 2050 could reach 14 million.

Given these trajectory statistics, the need for resources like Just Ask Dr. Macie; A Caregiver's Guide to Care, authored by Dr. Macie Smith, is immeasurable. Dr. Smith has the unique ability to teach families how to plan for their loved one's golden years while ensuring they enjoy the greatest quality of life possible.

In the pages that follow, Dr. Smith helps us to understand and work through what could be difficult situations that often accompany aging. She shows us it doesn't have to be stressful or problematic. The key is knowledge of the population and preparation for their needs; areas of which

Dr. Smith is expertly versed. Through her scholarly pursuits and practical application, Dr. Smith outlines for us a guide to caregiving that is loving and respectful of one's dignity; all at the same time.

TABLE OF CONTENTS

Frequently Asked Questions

Is there a difference between Alzheimer's and dementia?　1

How is Alzheimer's or Dementia diagnosed?　4

What are considered treatable types of dementia?　7

How do I get [mom] to drink more water?　11

Why do people living with dementia remember some things?

14

Why do people with dementia act like children?　16

How is dementia treated?　18

Why is mom cursing all the time?　21

How can I stop mom from lying?　23

How can I stop [dad] from behaving badly?　26

Glossary of Terms　35

Notes Page　37

About the Author

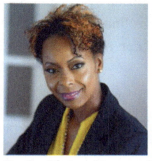

Dr. Macie P. Smith is an award-winning educator with 19 years of experience working with aging and vulnerable populations in South Carolina. She is the acting President of the National Association of Social Workers-South Carolina Chapter. Dr. Smith is a Licensed Social Worker, Certified Social Work Case Manager, and a Social Worker in Gerontology who provides private Geriatric Care Management to families living with dementia. She also serves as Professor and a Subject Matter Expert on the collegiate level in the areas of social work, social sciences, and public health at the University of South Carolina and the University of Phoenix.

Dr. Smith's work has been highlighted in several editions of University of Phoenix Faculty Matters Magazine for her continued contributions in the academic areas of teaching, discovery, integration, and application. She conducts research, develops programs, conducts program evaluations, and facilitates professional development training in the areas of health care management, human services development and program development. Her focus is coordinating quality care within aging and underserved communities.

Dr. Smith has a regular television segment on OnPoint on WACH FOX 57 entitled "Ask Dr. Macie." During her segment she answers health-related questions posed by viewers. She also pens a monthly column in the Carolina Panorama and has been a featured contributing writer in the All About Seniors Magazine.

Dr. Smith has been recognized as a 'Top 20 Under 40 Leader' by the South Carolina Black Pages Magazine for her work as a community and industry change agent. Dr. Smith's work has been featured on WACH FOX 57, WIS-TV's Awareness, WLTX, ABC Columbia, WFMV, WGCV, Alzheimer's Speaks radio, and WURD radio.

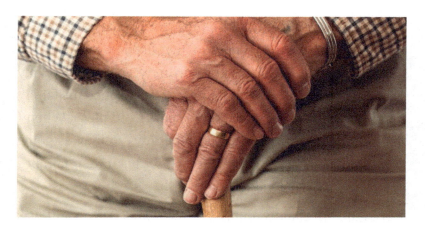

The Impetus Behind the Book

I've been working in the aging and disability arena since I was 22-years-old. I never would have dreamed that I still would be in this industry, educating others about how to engage and care for those who are living with a cognitive impairment. It wasn't until I was charged with the responsibility of ensuring the best quality of life for several seniors with dementia that I began to engulf myself in the research—getting extensive training in dementia-capable practices, both formally and informally.

Then it happened. In 2009, my paternal grandmother was diagnosed with Alzheimer's related dementia. This was one of the scariest times of my life, because after all the years of experience I had, I truly did not know what to do or who to call. My father and my sister were the primary caregivers for my grandmother and did a wonderful job; but we had moments where we struggled. I had to actually take off my granddaughter hat and put on my professional hat, because my grandmother, my dad, and my sister were now my clients. I did have the opportunity to resume my granddaughter role, but it was only after I trained my family and had all of my grandmother's services in place. When I took a moment to really assess what my family was going through, I couldn't help but realize what other families were, too, experiencing.

Here I am with many, many years of experience and I was at a loss; so, can you imagine the challenges of other families without my knowledge? I could not, in good faith, sit back and keep all the knowledge I had gained over the years to myself. I was on a mission to help other families by providing information, education, training, and care coordination. Therefore, I started my own business, Diversified Training Consultants Group.

Diversified Training Consultants Group is a training and geriatric care management business created to educate families while helping them navigate the long-term care system. Because of my passion to educate, I developed a dementia-capable curriculum for family caregivers entitled Dementia Speaks. Dementia Speaks has been conducted across the country in a host of communities. It is because of these community seminars and the one-on-one family contacts I've had over the years, that this book was created.

Along the way, I've been asked very similar questions about caring for someone with dementia. So, I thought, why not bundle the most popular questions in one place, provide my responses, and make available to everyone. That's what I've done here.

The goal of this publication is not to provide all the answers to your questions, but to offer some level of guidance for the continual care that will be required of someone living with dementia. Whether the person is living at home or in a residential community, they are going to need care and supervision. Everyone is different, however. What works for one, might not work for the other.

When you've met one person living with dementia, you've met that one person. Therefore, it is my intent that the information found in this book will be a blessing to those who find hope in the words written.

Introduction

There is a growing need to better support the more than 15 million family caregivers of those living with dementia. Family caregiving has been classified as a public health epidemic and so has dementia. As we sit contently reading this information, there are approximately 34 million family members currently providing caregiving support to those living with dementia. The type of support that is being provided is ongoing and never ceases, not even when the caregiver's health is failing. With many family caregivers passing away before the person with dementia, family caregivers need help and they need it now! So, here is my contribution to helping family caregivers everywhere; the nation's backbone to the long-term care system.

> *"Having Macie Smith provide instruction and access to information...is a huge advantage and a great example of how we seek to incorporate the most powerful voices in the caregiving community"*
>
> *Leeza Gibbons, Health Advocate/Journalist*

Included in this publication is a listing of questions that I am sure caregivers have found themselves asking on more than one occasion. I hope you find my candid responses not only helpful, but life-changing for you and those for whom you care.

Frequently Asked Questions:

Is there a difference between Alzheimer's and dementia?

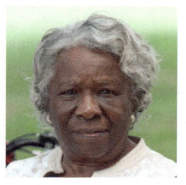

The fact that this question was asked led me to believe that lay persons are much savvier and more knowledgeable about the disease than ever before. This is huge for aging advocates and for professionals working in the industry. The knowledge and skillset that is gained over time will ultimately afford persons living with dementia and their families a better quality of life by way of information and education.

Yes, there is a difference between Alzheimer's disease and dementia. Dementia is not necessarily the diagnosis, although it is identified by a clinical code. Dementia is a group of behaviors or a set of symptoms that occurs as a result of a condition or conditions that are impairing one's thinking skills and/or cognitive abilities. It basically affects a person's ability to fully use their mental capacity; their mind. Some of the symptoms of a progressive form of dementia may include memory loss, forgetfulness, confusion and word-find difficulties (finding the right words to say in the right sentence). The symptoms could interfere with a person's social and occupational functioning. It could impair their ability to clearly communicate their needs and desires to others. It could also affect their ability to work through and complete simple tasks the way they used to, such as baking a cake or doing laundry.

There are several conditions that could cause dementia, including treatable conditions; but one of the most common causes of a progressive form of dementia is Alzheimer's disease. It is because of the popularity of Alzheimer's disease that the two terms, Alzheimer's and dementia, tend to be used interchangeably. And let's not forget about the all too popular term, "old timers", which is not a thing. The term "old timers" made its way into the discussion because age is the most common contributing factor in developing Alzheimer's. The largest segment of the population diagnosed with Alzheimer's or a progressive form of dementia is 65 years-old 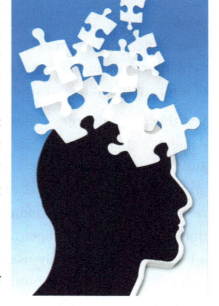 and older. Developing dementia or Alzheimer's is not a normal part of aging; however, age does increase the risk.

Alzheimer's is the actual disease that is progressive and irreversible. It is a brain disease that destroys brain cells and affects a person's memory, thinking skills, communication skills, and their ability to carry out simple activities of daily living, such as bathing; dressing; eating; toileting; walking; and swallowing.

Since Alzheimer's is, for now, progressive and irreversible there is no cure. So, the difference between Alzheimer's and dementia is that Alzheimer's is the disease and dementia is the symptoms of the disease process.

For example, if you went to the doctor because you had a sore throat and you were experiencing pain while swallowing, the doctor is going to assess the cause of your sore throat. Your diagnosis will not be "sore throat". Your diagnosis may be strep throat, a virus, sinus drainage, flu etc. So, whenever a person shows signs and symptoms of a medical or mental condition, you must figure out what's causing those symptoms. It is important to note here, too, that progressive forms of dementia are not a mental illness; it is a medical condition and should be treated as such.

How is Alzheimer's or Dementia diagnosed?

This question is often posed to me when individuals and families are questioning the diagnosis of Alzheimer's or dementia, which is a good thing. I often tell families not to accept a diagnosis of dementia or Alzheimer's at the first visit. If the doctor states that one has dementia, the first question that should be posed to the doctor is "What is causing the dementia?" Since dementia is caused by "something", this is a reasonable question.

A couple of dementia diagnoses one might hear of or see in medical records are Dementia NOS (not otherwise specified) and Dementia without Behavioral Disturbances. The only way to conclusively determine if a person has Alzheimer's is when an autopsy is performed. Since you can't get an autopsy while you're still living, doctors must rule out potential causes of dementia symptoms through a series of tests, both formal and informal. Ideally, the person should have a primary care physician (PCP) that will perform the following:

- Physical Examination
- Informant Questionnaire on Cognitive Decline
- Laboratory Tests

Once these tests are performed, the PCP should refer the person to a neurologist to have the following performed:

- Neurological Examination

- Brain Scans (i.e. MRI, PET, CAT)

- Cognitive Tests

After all tests have been performed and reviewed by each doctor, then the neurologist usually determines the diagnosis. All information should be shared with the primary care physician since he/she manages the person's overall care. Ensuring the primary care physician has all related medical documents increases comprehensive care and better health outcomes.

"My wife had reached the point as a result of a bad fall that I was seriously considering having to put her in a memory unit. Then we met Macie Smith. She recommended a plan with therapists, caregivers and other programs. As a result, my wife improved dramatically. We can certainly recommend Macie and her knowledge."

- Dementia Caregiver

When a dementia diagnosis is revealed to the patient, the first thing that should come out of the patient's mouth is "What type of dementia is it?" "What is causing me to experience dementia?" The medical professional should then assess what is causing the person's dementia symptoms (i.e. forgetfulness, memory loss, disorientation, agitation, anxiety, compulsiveness, irritability, aggression, etc).

Because I am a social worker and believe in reviewing all possible aspects of any life- changing occurrences, I highly encourage families to work with medical professionals to rule out all treatable causes of dementia, first.

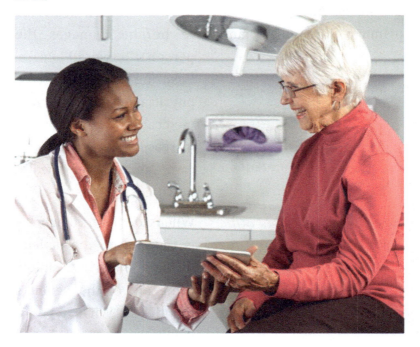

What are considered treatable types of dementia?

When I say "treatable" dementia, I mean that dementia is caused by a condition or situation that can be treated or addressed. Here is a list of areas that I tend to rule out before accepting a diagnosis of a progressive form of dementia, such as Alzheimer's:

#1 Medications. Has the person started taking a new medication? Are there any side effects to the medications they are taking? Are there any interactions or contraindications between the medications (i.e. are the medications fighting against each other)? Are the 5 rights being followed?

- The **Right** Person
- The **Right** Medication
- The **Right** Amount
- The **Right** Time
- The **Right** Route

I always encourage the use of one pharmacy; this way you can always go to the pharmacist to have a medication reconciliation performed to address potential issues with the medications prescribed. You simply ask the pharmacist to "check the medications for any adverse reactions." I tend to follow the path of least resistance here, as you will likely have a better chance of speaking with the pharmacist before you have the opportunity to schedule a talk with the person's physician.

#2 Infections. Does the person have a urinary tract infection (UTI)? A UTI is very common among the older population due to many reasons, but to name a few – they might not be as mobile as they used to be, they might not drink enough water or take in enough liquids, and they might be incontinent. You will want to request a urinalysis from a medical professional and have positive results prior to taking any antibiotics. In the event you would like to assess the likelihood of a UTI prior to seeing a medical professional, you can purchase a urinary screening kit from your local pharmacy. The kit is for "screening" purposes only and not a diagnostic tool. The test will only provide information that may suggest if the person might have a UTI. If the test is positive that means you should follow up with the physician as soon as possible.

#3 Dehydration. Is the person dehydrated? Because older adults and seniors tend to not drink a lot of water, the chances of dehydration occurring is very high. Dehydration can wreak havoc on a senior's psyche, if not treated. It can cause severe delirium, confusion, behavioral changes, and aggression. If you suspect dehydration, please seek medical attention immediately.

Note: One trip to the emergency room (ER) can land an older adult in the hospital with limited memory, limited inhibition, verbal and physical aggression, and hallucinations. This is what I call "hospital induced delirium". Delirium is a sudden state of confusion caused by various stimuli. When entering the halls of the emergency room/department there are many unwanted stimuli, such as the lighting; the noise; the people; and the procedures (prodding and poking with or without permission). When accessing the emergency room department for an acute condition, remember —the hospital staff is not familiar with the patient that is coming in for an emergent condition. Because of this, the senior may not receive a treatment plan best-suited for them. In most cases, this is the first and only time the hospitalist will have direct contact with this patient; therefore, the treatment provided is based on presenting symptoms, not necessarily the patient's history; the physician only knows what he/she is told and witnesses. So, you will want to share as much information as you can with the doctor about your loved one's history.

#4 Nutritional Imbalance. Is the person deprived of essential nutrients, such as vitamin B, vitamin D, or vitamin E? These vitamins are essential in maintaining optimal brain health. Therefore, you should have a medical professional complete laboratory tests to make the determination as to whether the person is lacking any essential vitamins. The lack of vitamin B12 is one area I tend to see a lot in the older population. If the person has vitamin B12 deficiency, the doctor might prescribe B12 tablets or even a B12 shot.

#5 Depression. Has there been a major life event, such as a death in the family? Is the person extremely sad about the death? If so, the person might be depressed. It might not be dementia at all. It is important to note that depression can be treated, even in older adults. But you have to report any life changes to the doctor, including irregular sleeping patterns or if they are not sleeping at all.

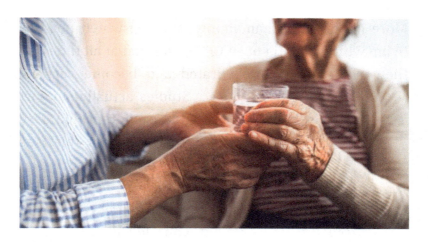

Mom doesn't like to drink water. How do I get her to drink more water?

Now, let's think about this. Who "reeeallly" likes to drink water?? We drink water because we know it's good for us and good for our body. But, many of us don't really like to drink water. Why? Because it doesn't have a taste and it makes you go to the bathroom. Well, let me be transparent, this is why I don't like drinking water and I know many of you feel the exact same way. Right? The truth of the matter is— people living with dementia don't like drinking water for the same exact reasons; it does not have a good taste and it causes them to have to go to the bathroom, A LOT. Since sweet is typically the last taste bud to go, they want to eat and drink things that have a good taste that they enjoy. So, why not make healthy items taste good.

More importantly than simply drinking water, persons living with dementia need to be hydrated at all times, so they won't become dehydrated and become very ill. Studies actually support that seniors could lose their sense of thirst as they age. Therefore, you have to be very creative when you're trying to get your loved one to stay hydrated.

"When I thought I'd come to the end of the road for help with my mother, Dr. Macie Smith stepped in and offered more avenues of health care for us to explore. She was a critical part of helping to facilitate her hospice care plan in the final stages of her battle with stage 4 pancreatic cancer. Because of Dr. Smith's contacts, impeccable char- acter and attention to detail I was able to obtain care for my mother that I didn't know was available. Having worked with her professionally and personally, I can say without a doubt she is among the best in her field of expertise."

~ Darci Strickland Rush, Journalist

You can try sweetening the water with natural sweeteners or try flavored water. You can try diluting the sweet beverage with water; in other words, "water it down." The key to this is to not let them see you"water down" their favorite beverage, because they might get mad at you (Just a little FYI that can save you some heartache). You can also try adding food items that are high in water content, such as fruits, jello, popsicles, yogurt, and ice cream. You can even simply remind them to drink; but it needs to be an invitation and not a command. You might say "Mom won't you come have a drink with me" as opposed to "Mom you need to drink something now." See the difference? The former is a little bit more inviting than the latter.

These tips are some ideas to help promote the hydration process. As you are ensuring proper hydration, please remain on the look out for water retention. If you see any indication of swelling, it might mean they are retaining too much fluid and you will want to seek medical attention right away.

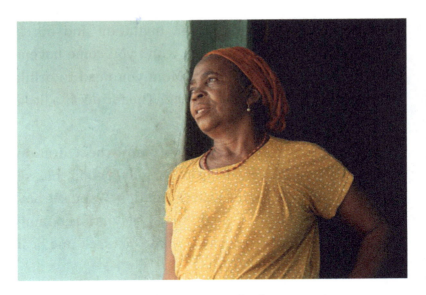

Why do people living with dementia remember some things but not other things?

This question is asked when families get a little flustered because the person with dementia can remember a long time ago, but experiences difficulty remembering recent events. For example, I had a client who could remember when she got married some 20 years ago, but experienced difficulty remembering when her daughter last visited her, which was the evening before.

The reason this happens is because Alzheimer's disease typically attacks the hippocampus early on in the disease process. The hippocampus is where your working memory/short term memory is stored. So, if the disease begins where the short term memories are formed, persons with Alzheimer's related dementia will experience difficulty remembering recent information. I like to say that the latest memory is the lost memory.

After storing information in the working/short term memory, a healthy brain pushes information through the executive functioning process and the information lands in the long-term memory; this is where the preserved memories are stored. So, there you have it!

Why do people with dementia act like children?

So, here's the thing, adults living with dementia often revert back to previous life's patterns. Notice, I did not say that they revert back to child-like behavior. Although a person living with dementia may begin to respond to his/her environment similar to that of a toddler, it does not make them a toddler or a child. They are simply doing the best they can with what they have. Just imagine how you respond to others when your mental faculties are impaired due to, I don't know, a medication that causes drowsiness. Because you are impaired, you might respond to things a little differently. For example, you might need someone to repeat things more than once because you couldn't quite get it the first time. You might become frustrated and irritated and lash out at people because of the side-effect of the medication. Well, people living with dementia respond the same way people living without dementia respond when their mental capacity is impaired. It doesn't make the two any different. In both situations the mental capacity is affected; however, one is only temporary, and the other is not. Guess which is which?

So, you see, people with dementia are people first and they deserve to be treated like the adults they are. When you begin to treat the symptoms, and not the person, the quality of life for the person and the caregiver diminishes greatly. For children, we do things to them and for them in order to teach them. But, for adults living with dementia, we are to prepare the environment with them in order to preserve their dignity and independence for as long as feasibly possible.

In order to be successful preparing the environment with them, we have to know who they were before they developed dementia. What did they like? What did they dislike? What activities did they enjoy doing? For my grandmother, she enjoyed fishing. So, we made sure she still could participate in the "fishing" process. When she could no longer go out in the boat to fish, we would catch the fish and bring the fish back to her house so that we could all clean the fish together. She enjoyed that because it was an important part of her life and it made her feel valuable that she still could participate in her own life decisions. This was made possible because we prepared her environment with her by understanding the joys of her life.

As you begin to prepare the environment with your loved one, please remember them as a person and not as a disease. They still are human and value their dignity, identity, and independence; celebrate who they are not the condition they have.

How is dementia treated?

Dementia can be treated, but only for a period of time. Alzheimer's disease cannot be treated. Dementia is treated with medications that addresses the symptoms (memory loss, confusion, forgetfulness, etc). As the disease progresses, the medications may delay the progression of dementia for some time. This allows the person living with dementia to have a longer quality of life. For example, they might forget their daughter's name, but they know that person is their daughter. As the disease and dementia progresses, now the person thinks their daughter is their mother because the daughter looks exactly like the person's mother from years ago. If the medication is given early enough, this type of progression could be delayed or slowed.

When it comes to treatment, I highly recommend families study and have accessible the Beers Criteria Checklist. This is a comprehensive medication list that was developed by the American Geriatrics Society that provides guidance to families caring for older adults or seniors. All too often, the family is treated and not the patient. Medical professionals tend to prescribe medications for the family as opposed to the person living with dementia. What I mean by this is, families request medications to address the behaviors of the person living with dementia. Behavioral health medications, along with pain medications and muscle relaxants could have harmful effects on the geriatric population. In fact, The American Geriatrics Society warns of many different medications that the geriatric population should avoid or use with caution. The use of the medications outlined in the checklist should be discussed with one's physician to assess the benefits and the risks. For clarity, the geriatric population consists of those age 65 and older. Working with this population is a specialty area; therefore, if you have an opportunity to work with a Geriatrician, you would want to make that a priority.

Because there is not a cure for Alzheimer's, I foster, encourage, and promote non-prescription therapy. Being able to prepare an environment where the person with dementia can feel alive, happy, and have a sense of belonging is of the utmost importance. One of the ways this can be achieved is through music; playing the music that is representative of the prime of their life. You know that music that you play when you want to reminisce about the good 'ole days? They like to reminisce about the good 'ole days, as well. You will want to do an Internet search, ask them, or ask those who are close in age to the person with dementia to narrow down the type of music they might like to hear. Once you begin to play the music, watch for non-verbal signs of enjoyment, such as tapping of the feet; nodding of the head; swaying of the shoulders; widening of the eyes;

"I admire you...and my gratitude for the education of a lifetime!"

-Aging Professional

smiling; laughing; and excitable vocals. These are indications that they are loving it!

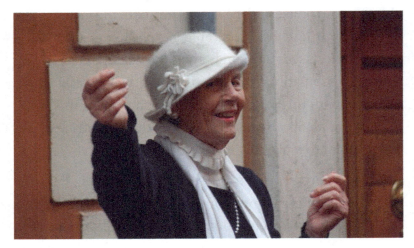

Why is mom cursing all the time? She's never cursed.

I respond to this question by stating, "Your mom has known you all of your life, you have not known your mom all of her life." You might not have known your mom to curse; but she probably used to curse back in the day. Keep in mind, we learn those bad words in grade school, early on in life. So, as your mom journeys through the disease process, she will remember those words and will use them on occasion. But she is using these words for one reason and one reason only; to get your attention. She has an unmet need that is not being addressed.

When we learned bad words as a child, we knew not to say them because we did not want to get in trouble; we knew what the consequences might have been. Since you cannot hear, see, taste, touch, or smell "consequences" they do not exist to someone with dementia. Those living with dementia become very concrete thinkers as the disease progresses; therefore, the things that are not tangible to them are not tolerable by them. Because the brain is deteriorating, persons living with dementia use the words they can understand and what they can most successfully project; it affords them the ability to take back control of their life.

You also must consider that the ability to control thoughts, responses, and reactions are slowly fading. They are becoming more and more uninhibited as the disease progresses; what they think, is what they say. What comes up in their mind, comes out of their mouth.

The reason this occurs is because consequences are not concrete ideas; therefore, they don't exist. People with dementia begin to think more concretely as the disease progresses as opposed to abstractly. In their concrete thinking, they are unable to think beyond what they see. An abstract-thinker is able to problem-solve and use appropriate reasoning for various things. For example, an abstract-thinker understands that a bouquet of roses is decoration for the table; a concrete thinker views the bouquet of roses as flowers that must be planted and watered in the ground. It is because of this thinking pattern that consequences are meaningless to them. Since you can't see, touch, taste, or smell "consequences" it is unrealistic to them; thereby, not an essential factor.

How can I stop mom from lying?

I often begin by saying, "What do you mean by lying?" What's reality to a person living with dementia, may not be reality to a person without dementia. If a person with dementia believes that you stole their money, then that is what is 100% real to them. If it is real to them, for you to be a successful caregiver, it has to be real to you, as well.

My grandmother felt that someone was stealing her pots on a weekly basis. She felt it so much so that she would call the police to have the person arrested. Fortunately for us (her family), she did not know exactly who the person was stealing her pots. She became fearful, depressed, and upset that someone would come into her home and steal her pots. I would see my grandmother go through these streams of emotions about a situation that was an actual occurrence in her life; but it was not real...to us. Because I saw the toll it was taking on her health and her soul, I developed the VCR approach and shared it with my family so that we all could be on the same page when communicating with her about those pots. VCR stands for validate, comfort, and redirect. Once you begin the VCR approach, you will need to do it over and over again for consistency and success.

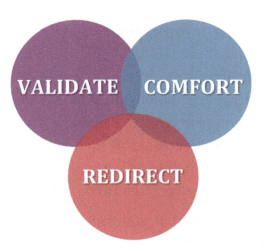

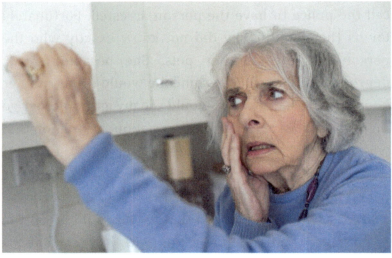

Validate. I validated my grandmother by telling her that I understood what she was feeling because it had happened to me in the past. Someone had also stolen from me and it hurt me to my heart.

Comfort. I offered comfort to my grandmother by telling her that everything would be okay. I would help protect her and her possessions by visiting more often.

Redirect. I redirected her concerning thoughts by coaching her to physically move from the location where she was visibly upset to a location that was pleasing to her. Because my grandmother loved to raise chickens, I would redirect the conversation and began talking about chickens laying eggs. This conversation would move us from the den area to the backyard where she raised chickens. From that point on, she forgot about the lady stealing her pots...until the next day, that is. When the conversation resurfaced about the pots the next day, we would VCR all over again.

Validate   Comfort   Redirect

Dad won't allow me to do anything for him. He acts out so bad when I attempt to do for him. How can I stop him from behaving badly?

My first thought is, "How does an adult act out?" Families use this term to define challenging, sometimes uncontrollable behaviors. I, wholeheartedly, understand the concerns from families when their loved ones are behaving in a manner that is potentially dangerous for them and those around them. More times than not, it is the way in which we communicate with them that sets the stage for their responses. Negative interactions beget negative responses.

Check out this list of communication tips I compiled for you from the acronym B.R.E.A.T.H.E. Breathe is an appropriate acronym when you're discussing dementia caregiving. Because the cost of caring is identifiable through physical, emotion, and spiritual perils, you must take a moment to breathe and to think about your next steps, and what they should look like. It is my hope that when you take a moment to BREATHE, you will think about these steps:

B. Be. Be who they want you to be at that moment. Have you ever thought about being an actor or actress? Now is your time. As the disease progresses, they might view you as their parent as opposed to their children.

DO NOT correct them. Be who they need you to be at that moment. Play the role you are given.

R. Reassurance. Provide reassurance at any moment in which they are fearful. You must remember that they were aware of what was going on with them before anyone else noticed. They are afraid of losing their mind. And that is actually what is transpiring. You would do for them what you would want someone to do for you. Tell them that everything is going to be okay and begin to redirect them to a point of conversation or activity that is more pleasurable. This involves physically guiding them to a different place in the home or environment to get their mind off of what's worrisome (which is what we did with my grandmother).

E. Empathy. Practice empathy. They don't want you to feel sorry for them. They want your help! You will want to better understand that they are trying to hold on to the fibers of their being with everything they have. The part of their body that manages who they are and what they do (their mind) is deteriorating. They are doing the best they can with what they have. Continue to speak to the heart and soul of the person. Don't give life to the disease by making their condition the pinnacle point of your engagement with them. They don't need continual reminders of their limitations. It's not about what they can no longer do. But what is it that you can do to help them maintain their dignity, identity, and independence throughout the disease process?

A. Allow. Allow them to express themselves in the manner in which they can at the moment. Allow them the opportunity to do for themselves. I know you don't like it when dad puts on a blue shirt with brown pants. But it's not about you. It's about him and what he is able to do for himself. If your discussion points begin with "I" and end with "me" then it's about you, not them. If it's not harmful to them or others; if it is not dangerous or bothersome to them or others allow them to do it. I know you heard the old saying, "Pick your battles." Well, this is what I'm telling you to do. Just let it go. No harm-No hindrance.

T. Talk. Keep the dialogue going with the person who has dementia. There will come a time when they might not be able to communicate effectively with comprehensible words, but they will always have the ability to communicate. Sure, the caregiver is responsible for both sending and understanding the messages for the person living with dementia. Sure, the person with dementia may have poor ability to use verbal messages and prefers non-verbal messages, instead. Sure, the person with dementia will require that communication is broken down into step-by-step instructions. Although their communication may not be based on reality, they still can communicate. They communicate through words, expressions, body language, and touch. You should begin to adjust your communication-style to fit their needs.

Again, it's not about you; it's about them. They cannot change, but you can.

I would be lying if I said that communicating with someone with dementia would not be challenging, because it will be. Nevertheless, here are a few additional tips that could help you continue to engage the person throughout the disease journey.

1. Be patient, speak slowly, and allow them time to respond to your question or statement.

2. Don't overload them with questions. Ask one question at a time.

3. Check for hearing loss. Loss of hearing just might be the reason they are not engaging with you, because they didn't hear you.

4. Show interest in what they are talking about even if you have heard it several times. If they are asking repeated questions, answer them and/or write it down. They might not have remembered that they even asked you the question. Repetition can be an indication of pain, fear, or distress. It can also be a sign of strength and power. This might be the only form of communication they can remember, so they do it often and independently; thereby, regaining their power.

5. Avoid criticism and/or correcting. Do not argue or confront them. Have you ever argued with

someone with dementia? Did you win? Probably not. When you argue with someone, you are trying to change their mind. The mind of a person living with dementia is constantly changing without any help from you. If their communication is not based on reality, then step into their reality and play the role. I know you might be saying, "But what if mom is accusing me of stealing her money?" Or, "What if she still thinks she can drive her car, but has had several accidents?"

Try these tips on for size:

a. Accept blame and let her know that whatever it is she is accusing you of, it was to help her or someone she loves and provide reassurance along the way. (For example, if she says, "You stole my money!" You say, "I am sorry. I had to purchase your medication so that your leg will heal so that you can make it to your weekly hair appointment."

b. Have duplicates of the item she is accusing you of stealing, so you can replace the "stolen" item.

c. DO NOT say that what she is saying is not true. You are basically calling her a liar and that is not going to work out well at all.

d. If she wants to drive her car, DO NOT treat her like a child and restrict her. But don't allow her to drive, either. Instead, allow her to make the decision not to drive. Try disabling the car without her knowing so that it won't crank. She might then say, "I need for the tow truck to come pick up the car to take it in for fixing." BINGO! Out of sight, out of mind. She made her own decision to remove the car; no one made it for her. Once the car leaves the house to go to the shop; the car will ALWAYS be in the shop. You know what I mean?

H. Humor. Do use humor, but not at the person's expense. Do not make jokes about them without them. Laugh together about what they feel is comical. Laughter is good for the soul, even when a person has dementia. My motto is, "If you're not laughing, you're crying." So why not find the joy in the here and now. Trust me, there are going to be things to appropriately laugh about.

E. Establish. Establish a routine. Establishing a routine is so vitally important to the person with dementia and important to their caregiver(s), as well. When a routine is established with the person in mind, they can continue to do things independently and not have to think about it. For example, how many steps are involved in brushing your teeth? I'll wait...chances are, you don't know off the top of your head, but you can do it successfully because of the routine you've established for brushing your teeth. This is called remote memory or muscle memory; you remember by doing and so does the person living with dementia.

In following their lead, if they normally wake up at 10:00am, then that is their routine. They might know exactly what to do next (i.e. bathe, brush their teeth, eat breakfast) if they wake up the same time every day. But if the routine is interrupted (i.e. an 8:00am doctor's appointment), they might have a bad day because they cannot quite figure out what to do next. This could cause increased confusion, anxiety, and irritability. A person with dementia has difficulty coping with change and new information. Therefore, having a structured routine allows the person with dementia the opportunity to maintain his/her abilities, and it will save you time, energy, and anguish.

> *"When our mom was diagnosed with Dementia, we were thrust head and heart first into (for us) a new world of mental illness and forced to navigate the incredibly complicated healthcare system. Then we met Dr. Macie Smith and through her class (Dementia Speaks) we were able to find solid, reliable and accurate guidance in caring for our loved one."*
>
> *-Tanya Rodriguez-Hodges*

And there you have it! This is my list of the most commonly asked questions regarding dementia-capable care. I do hope you were able to relate to some of what was written here. Take this book with you and refer to it along the way. It will be a long journey, but you won't have to go through it alone. There are support groups out there that are just waiting for your call.

You also can visit my You Tube page "Ask Dr. Macie" for pointers 24/7. Although there is not a cure for Alzheimer's disease and other progressive forms of dementia, there is care; your care.

Now, I say to each of you, just BREATHE and watch how life changes begin to unfold for the better, for you and the person with dementia.

Take the BREATHE challenge, today!

Take care.

"Thanks again for an awesome training! The information was impactful both professionally and personally. I came home and gave my sister a BIG kiss! I've already used what I learned and she is responding wonderfully.

Amazing."

- Dementia Caregiver

Glossary of Terms

Adverse /ad´vers /
Unfavorable and potentially harmful

Autopsy /´ô, täpsē/
An examination of body or organ after death

Cognitive Tests
A test that examines such areas as memory, orientation, reasoning, and numerical

**Contraindication \kän-tre-, in-de-'kä-shen **
When medication and/or medical treatment cause harm

Executive Functioning
The brain's ability to retrieve, encode, and store information for long-term use

Geriatric
Population of individuals age 65+

Hippocampus /hipe' kampes/
The part of the brain where short term memories are formed

Informant Questionnaire on Cognitive Decline
The person who provides the doctor information on the type of symptoms the patient is displaying

Incontinent /in'känt(e)nent/
Having no control or insufficient control over bowel and/or bladder

Irreversible /,i(r)re'verseb(e)l/
Unable to return back to the original state

Primary Care Physician (PCP)
The main doctor that manages all medical conditions

Progressive /pre'gresiv/
Gets worse over time and in stages

Psyche /'sīkē/
A person's mind

Reminiscence /reme'nisens/
Remembering enjoyable events that occurred in the past

Side Effects
Unfavorable or harmful symptoms occurring as a result of taking medications or receiving medical treatment

Uninhibited /ene'hibeded/
Expressing feelings without regard for anything or anyone, unrestricted views and opinions

Urinalysis /yo˘ore'naleses/
A urine test

Notes Page

Notes Page

Notes Page

Notes Page

Notes Page

Notes Page

Notes Page

Notes Page

Notes Page

Notes Page

Notes Page

Notes Page

Notes Page

Notes Page

Notes Page

Notes Page

Notes Page

Notes Page

Notes Page

Notes Page